Blood Pressure

Learn how to reduce high blood pressure and control low blood pressure with and without medication

By KG | PHYSIO

© 2016 KG | PHYSIO

All rights reserved. No portion of this book may be reproduced in any form without permission from the publisher, except as permitted by UK copyright law.

Disclaimer: This book is not intended as a substitute for the medical advice of physicians. The reader should regularly consult a physician in matters relating to his/her health, and particularly with respect to any symptoms that may require medical diagnosis or medical attention.

Cover by Kane Georgiou.

Table of Contents

Introduction 1

Chapter One: What You Need to Know about Blood Pressure............ 6

    What exactly is high blood pressure? 6

    How is blood pressure measured? 7

    High Blood Pressure (Hypertension) 9

        What are the causes of high blood pressure? 9

        Are there symptoms or warning signs of high blood pressure? 10

        How can high blood pressure affect your health? 11

    Low Blood Pressure (Hypotension) 12

        Causes of Low Blood Pressure 12

        Are there any symptoms or warning signs of low blood pressure (hypotension)? 13

        How can low blood pressure affect your health? 14

Chapter Two: How to regulate your blood pressure with medication 16

    Managing High Blood Pressure with Prescription Medications 17

Chapter Three: Managing Low Blood Pressure 32

Chapter Four: How to Manage Blood Pressure without Medication 36

    Diet... 37

    Exercise.. 45

Chapter Five: Using Meditation and/or Yoga to help regulate your blood pressure 50

Chapter SIX: Tips to Control your Blood Pressure 63

Conclusion 67

Appendix 1: Glossary of terms: 69

Appendix II: References 70

Preview of 'Meditation for Beginners' 79

Introduction

There are many things that can go wrong with our health as we age and blood pressure is one of them. What exactly is blood pressure? What is the difference between high blood pressure (hypertension) and low blood pressure (hypotension)? How can it be controlled?

We shall answer these as well as many other questions concerning blood pressure health in this eBook. This is not a medical journal entry filled with confusing medical terminology, but rather an informative guide, written in everyday language to help provide some insight into the most commonly asked questions and other concerns regarding blood pressure health. This eBook is not meant as a diagnostic tool for either high or low blood pressure. If you feel that might be suffering from either, you need to get a professional medical diagnosis. This eBook is meant simply as a guide to provide you with some helpful information.

A diagnosis with hypertension is not the end of the world. Yes, it is a serious health concern and should not be taken lightly, by any means. However, blood pressure can be regulated through medication, change in diet, exercise and simple lifestyle changes. This eBook will give you some helpful information on the various types of medication that are available for hypertension, as well as some other things you can do to improve your blood pressure rate. We shall also discuss how to raise low blood pressure.

Again, the purpose of this eBook is again for educational purposes only. You should discuss any medication, diet or lifestyle changes such as exercise with your physician.

In the first chapter we give the definition of blood pressure as well as the risk factors, causes, symptoms and possible health risks of both high and low blood pressure. We will tell you the difference between systolic and diastolic blood pressure as well as how blood pressure readings are calculated and interpreted. We shall discuss some of the causes and factors that may place you at risk for high or low blood pressure respectively.

In chapter two we shall take a look at the medications that are often prescribed for high blood pressure, as well as the possible side effects of each. It is important that you disclose your full medical history and openly and honestly answer any questions your physician may ask you as these will help determine what type of medication is best for you. The medications that we shall discuss in this chapter are the following:

- **Aldosterone Receptor Antagonists**
- **Alpha Blockers**
- **Alpha Beta Blockers**
- **Angiotensin II Receptor Blockers (ARBs)**
- **Angiotensin-Converting Enzyme (ACE) Inhibitors**
- **Beta Blockers**

- **Calcium Channel Blockers**
- **Central-Acting Agents**
- **Diuretics**
- **Renin Inhibitors**
- **Vasodilators**

Don't let the medical terminology throw you off. There are various generic types for each of the above and your doctor will take a detailed medical history before prescribing one of the above medications. Every case is different and you may be prescribed one or more of the above medications, or something different altogether. You may not even need medication or you may just need to take it for a short time. Or you may need to take it for the rest of your life. Do not judge your specific case by anyone else's as everyone's chemical and genetic makeup is different, as well as other circumstance such as lifestyle and other health concerns. Listen to what your physician tells you and follow their advice to the letter.

We will also offer some insights into some of the most common vitamins and herbal supplements that are often prescribed in addition to medication. Again, this is not a complete list and you should only add vitamins or other supplements to your daily regime after discussing them first with your primary care physician or specialist.

In Chapter Three, we shall take a closer look at hypotension or low blood pressure. While low blood pressure is somewhat easier to manage than high blood pressure, it is not to be taken lightly as it may be an indicator of an underlying medical issue (which we will discuss in detail in Chapter 2) In Chapter Three we shall discuss some ways you can naturally raise your blood pressure.

In Chapter 4 we shall take a close look at how diet and exercise can help regulate your blood pressure. The DASH Diet was specially designed for lowering and regulating blood pressure and we shall give a detailed description of the DASH Diet as well as recommended foods for those who are to follow this diet. Again, any dietary changes should be discussed with your doctor.

We shall also take a look at how regular physical exercise can help control your blood pressure rate. Of course you should ever start any type of physical exercise without first discussing it with your doctor.

In Chapter 5 we shall discuss how relaxation therapy can help regulate your blood pressure, specially meditation and yoga.

Mediation, particularly Mindfulness Meditation is extremely effective at helping to lower and ultimately control your blood pressure. We shall discuss how mediation can help control your blood pressure as well as a brief guide on how to practice Mindfulness Meditation, as well as how to incorporate Mindfulness into your everyday life to help regulate your blood pressure on a daily basis.

Yoga is also another extremely effective way to help lower and regulate blood pressure. Yoga, like meditation, has been around for centuries, and is becoming increasingly popular as a relaxation technique in today's hectic, fast-paced society. We shall give you some insights into how yoga can help regulate your blood pressure as well as 5 of the top recommended cardiovascular yoga positions and how to achieve these positions.

In the final chapter we shall offer some other helpful tips on how to control your blood pressure such as reducing your salt intake, eliminating stress from your life and cutting back on caffeine. It might seem like a lot, but these changes can greatly impact your blood pressure levels.

Then we shall come to a conclusion and include a small glossary of terms as well as the references that were used in writing this eBook.

So pull up a chair, pour yourself a cup of green tea, munch on some raw veggies and relax. We hope that you find this eBook to be very informative and that it answers some of the questions you may be asking yourself. The advice in this book is not definite; again, you need to discuss your individual situation with your doctor. Rather this book is an overall guide to provide you some insight into controlling your blood pressure and achieving a happier and healthier lifestyle.

CHAPTER ONE

What You Need to Know about Blood Pressure

So you have recently be diagnosed with high blood pressure and you're at a loss. How did this happen to me? How will this affect my health, And my life?

High blood pressure is extremely common as thousands of people are diagnosed with high blood pressure every year. While it is cause of concern, it is not a death sentence. In this chapter we shall take a look at what causes high blood pressure as well as the symptom. But first it's important to understand exactly what blood pressure is and what it means to our health. In the following section, we shall discuss how our blood pressure affects our bodies.

What exactly is high blood pressure?

As our heart beats it pumps blood throughout our bodies to supply it with oxygen and energy. As the blood is traveling through our blood vessels, it pushed against the side. The strength at which it pushes against the walls of our blood vessels is known as blood pressure. Blood pressure is responsible for distributing white blood cells, antibodies and certain hormones like insulin. As our blood is distributed throughout our bodies it is able to help rid the body of toxic waste products as well as the toxins in our kidney and liver.

High blood pressure occurs when there is additional strain placed on the heart and blood pressure, which causes them to become weakened or damaged. Low blood pressure occurs when the blood pressure is lower than normal. Normal blood pressure is usually read between 90/60 mmHG and 120/80 mmHg. When you have a low blood pressure reading it means that your heart and brain are not getting enough oxygen. Both high and low blood pressure can be extremely harmful if not treated properly.

How is blood pressure measured?

Blood pressure is measured by an instrument called a sphygmomanometer, which was invented mid 1800's. It reads how much an arterial pressure is needed before the pulse in our arms stops for a brief time. If you have been to a doctor's office or had any type of medical examination in your lifetime, you are familiar with getting your blood pressure take. The instrument consists of a cuff, rubber armband and a machine or hand pump that that applies the pressure and measures the reading. The nurse, nurse practitioner, physician's assistant or doctor will also use a stethoscope to listen to the blood as it flows through one of your arteries. They will inflate the cuff to determine your systolic blood pressure. The "whooshing" sound that is hard though the stethoscope as is deflates is your systolic blood pressure. After this noise has subsided, this indicates your diastolic blood pressure.

Systolic blood pressure, the top number on your reading, is the higher number and measures the pressure of your arteries when the heart muscles contract (aka your heartbeat). Diastolic blood pressure measures the pressure when the heart is resting between heartbeats, while the blood refills. Blood pressure is measured in millimeters of mercury or mmHG, for example a reading of "120/80mm Hg) means that your systolic blood pressure is 120 mmHg and your diastolic blood pressure is 80 mmHg.

Below is a chart for determining low vs high blood pressure in adults.

\multicolumn{3}{c	}{JNC 7 Blood Pressure Classification In Adults Aged ≥ 18 Years}
Category	Systolic	Diastolic
Normal	<120 and	<80
Prehypertension	120-139 or	80-89
Hypertension, Stage 1	140-159 or	90-99
Hypertension, Stage 2	≥160 or	≥100

National Heart, Lung, and Blood Institute. *JNC 7 Express. The Seventh Report of the Joint National Committee on the Prevention, Detection, Evaluation and Treatment of High Blood Pressure. 2003.*

Image source: *http://blood-pressurechart.blogspot.com/p/blood-pressure-chart.html*

You should get your blood pressure taken during your yearly visit with your primary care physician. They will determine if it falls in the normal range. If not, they will then diagnose which type of blood pressure disorder you have and will advise you as to how it can be treated. High blood pressure is also known as hypertension, and is more common as it affects up to 20% of adults over the age of 18. Low blood pressure, also known as hypotension, is anything below 120/80 and while less common, can be serious as it often an indicator of another underlying medical condition

In the next section we will take a look at the causes, symptoms and health factors of both high and low blood pressure.

High Blood Pressure (Hypertension)

What are the causes of high blood pressure?

While the exact causes of high blood pressure are not medically proven at this time, there are several risk factors that may contribute to hypertension. They are listed below:

- Overweight or obesity
- Too much salt in your diet
- Lack of physical exercise or activity
- stress and anxiety
- Chronic kidney disease
- High consumption of Alcoholic beverages (more than 2 drinks per day)
- Genetics
- Family History
- Aging
- Thyroid disorders
- Sleep apnea

- Adrenal disorders
- Too much fat content in diet
- Diabetes
- Smoking

Certain prescription medications may contribute to hypertension as well, including birth control pills, and asthma medications as well as hormone or estrogen therapies. Certain over-the counter medications such as allergy, flu or cold relief medications can also affect your blood pressure. Medications can affect the way your body controls salt and fluid levels which can cause your blood vessels to constrict, thus creating hypertension.

Are there symptoms or warning signs of high blood pressure?

Contrary to what people may say, there are rarely any visible or physical warning signs of hypertension (high blood pressure) which is why it is often called "the silent killer." This is why it is important to monitor your blood pressure regularly if you have been diagnosed with hypertension. Unfortunately, by the time symptoms start to show, the victim is usually already in crisis. Symptoms don't normally show until the systolic blood pressure is over 180 mmHg and diastolic blood pressure is over 100 mmHg. Anytime you blood pressure reading is this high for either your systolic or diastolic blood pressure, you need to seek immediate medical attention.

Some of the symptoms that you may experience if you are expressing Stage 2 Hypertension are as follows:

- Shortness of breath

- Nosebleeds
- Severe tension headaches
- Uncontrollable anxiety

If you are experiencing secondary hypertension you need to seek immediate medical care as it can result in the following complications

- Brain swelling or bleeding
- Tear in the main artery of the heart
- Heart attack
- Fluid in the heart of lungs
- Stroke
- Seizures (mainly in pregnant women who have with Preeclampsia)

How can high blood pressure affect your health?

The higher your blood pressure, the more you are at risk for serious health issues. Below are some of the serious medical conditions that are caused by hypertension:

- Heart attack
- Heart failure
- Stroke
- Dementia
- Peripheral arterial disease (which could result in loss of limbs)
- Diabetes
- Arterial Scholaris
- Kidney Damage

- Vision Loss
- Angina
- Fluid in the lungs, heart or brain
- Blood clots
- Erectile Dysfunction
- Aneurysm
- Coronary Artery Disease
- Kidney Failure
- Enlarged Heart

Low Blood Pressure (Hypotension)

Causes of Low Blood Pressure

As previously stated, there are several medical conditions that can cause low blood pressure. These are as follows:

- Pregnancy
- Endocrine issues
- Heart issues
- Loss of blood
- Dehydration
- Anaphylactic shock
- Other severe allergic reactions
- Poor nutrition
- Vitamin deficiencies
- Infections
- Hypoglycemia
- Heat exhaustion or heat stroke
- Hormonal issues

- High body temperature
- Sepsis (blood infection)
- Low body temperature
- Liver disease

Just as with hypertension, certain medications can contribute to low blood pressure. These include water pills, alpha and/or beta blockers, certain antidepressants, drugs used to treat Parkinson's disease and certain heart medications.

Are there any symptoms or warning signs of low blood pressure (hypotension)?

Low blood pressure often indicates another underlying health issues, especially as many of the symptoms of hypertension are similar to other health conditions.

Some of the common symptoms of hypotension include:

- Fainting
- Dizziness, lightheadedness or vertigo
- Difficulty concentrating
- Cold or clammy hands
- Pale skin
- Blurred vision
- Shallow and rapid breathing
- Extreme thirst
- Dehydration
- Nausea and vomiting
- Fatigue
- Depression

How can low blood pressure affect your health?

Hypotension is often an indicator of other underlying medical conditions. Hypotension can be caused by so many different factors, as indicated above including dehydration, heat exhaustion and standing up too quickly. Most times, your blood pressure will return to normal within a few minutes. However, if you are experiencing frequent bouts of low blood pressure, it could be an indicator of another medical condition:

- Kidney failure
- Diverticulitis
- Anemia
- Vertigo
- Diabetes
- Pregnancy
- Congestive Heart Failure
- Internal Bleeding
- Deep Vein Thrombosis
- Dehydration
- Sepsis
- Kidney Infection
- Angina
- Heat Stroke
- Stroke
- Shock
- Aneurysm
- Heart Attack
- Staph Infection
- Atrial Fibrillation

- Pancreatitis
- Toxic Shock Syndrome
- Anorexia
- Bulimia

Conclusion

So as you can see, both hypertension and hypotension can be causes for concern. However, if diagnosed properly and early, they can both be treated. There are medications available to help regulate both high and low blood pressure. However, there are also other ways you can regulate your blood pressure such as change in diet, exercise and herbal supplements. In the following chapters we shall discuss ways to treat and regulate your blood pressure. Simple things like reducing your salt intake and moderate exercise can greatly improve your blood pressure rate. Relaxation exercises such as yoga and meditation can also help control your blood pressure.

CHAPTER TWO

How to regulate your blood pressure with medication

There are plenty of medication options for those who need to control their blood pressure. Your doctor will take a detailed history of your health and decide which medication works best for you. Ideally, it would be better if you did not have to rely on medication to regulate your blood pressure levels, but unfortunately, it some cases it cannot be avoided. However with proper diet and exercise, as well as some other lifestyle changes, you may eventually be able to stop the medication. Again, this must all be discussed with your physician as this is a serious health issue and not to be taken lightly. We shall discuss some alternatives to medication later, but in this chapter we shall focus on the different types of medication you can take to help control your blood pressure.

Managing High Blood Pressure with Prescription Medications

Your doctor will determine if you need to treat your hypertension with prescription medication. They will perform a thorough medical exam, possibly perform some routine tests and take a blood and/or urine sample. You will have to provide a detailed medical and family history, including all prior and current health conditions, surgeries or other procedures and history (if any) of alcohol or substance abuse. You will need to disclose any and all medications, prescription or otherwise, as well as any herbal supplements or vitamins that you are taking, as well as any allergies or other health issues or concerns you may have.

While prescription medication may be initially required to help lower your blood pressure, it might only be for a short time. Or it could be a lifelong occurrence. Of course, the final say is up to your doctor. However, if you are able to make changes to your diet and lifestyle that can aid in lowering your blood pressure naturally, you may be able to stop taking prescription medications. However, it is important to remember that every case is different and the final say is to be made by your primary care physician or specialist.

There are many kinds of medications and of course the information can be very overwhelming, and extremely scientific. And not all of us have medical degrees, so for the purpose of this eBook, we shall keep it simple and give just a general guide as to the most common types of medication, along with basic information and the side effects of each.

1. Aldosterone Receptor Antagonists

What are aldosterone antagonists?
Aldosterone receptors antagonists help rid the body of extra water and act as a diuretic. They also work extremely well at helping the body retain potassium so in essence they can help regulate blood pressure.

What are the possible side effects of aldosterone antagonists?

Mild
- Nausea
- Vomiting
- Stomach cramps
- Diarrhea

Moderate
- Dizziness
- Hives

Severe
- Breathing issues
- Irregular heartbeat
- Numbness in extremities (hands, feet)
- Tingling in face and lips
- Swelling in face, lips, tongue or throat
- Confusion

As with any medication, seek immediate medical help if you experience any severe or adverse side effects from this medication.

2. Alpha Blockers

What are alpha blockers?

Alpha blockers help relax certain muscles in the body and can aid in helping to keep blood vessels open by preventing norepinephrine (or noradrenalin) from managing the muscles in the veins and smaller parties tighten, thus helping to lower and regulate blood pressure.

What are the possible side effects of alpha blockers?

Mild
- Dizziness
- Lethargy
- Nausea
- Headaches

Moderate
- Swelling in ankles or legs
- Sleep disturbances

Severe
- Rash

If you experience any of the moderate to severe side effects when taking alpha blockers, or any other adverse effects, please seek immediate medical care.

3. Alpha Beta Blockers

What are alpha beta blockers?

Alpha beta blockers are similar to beta blockers (see below) but are normally prescribed for those are at risk for heart failure as well as high blood pressure.

What are the possible side effects of alpha beta blockers?

Mild
- Headache
- Weight gain
- Diarrhea

Moderate
- Dizziness
- Dry or itchy eyes

Severe
- Shortness of breath
- Heart palpitations

Seek immediate medical attention if you suffer from severe or adverse side effects from this medication.

4. Angiotensin II Receptor Blockers (ARBs)

What are Angiotensin II receptor blockers?
ARBs assist in relaxing the blood vessels by blocking the angiotensin from acting to narrow the blood vessels. This will make it much easier for your blood to flow through the blood vessels. Thus reducing your blood pressure levels, also ARB's aid in increasing the release of sodium and water into the urine as opposed to the bloodstream, which also aids in lowering blood pressure.

What are the sides affects of Angiotensin II receptor blockers?

Mild
- Dizziness

- Sinus issues (stuffy or runny nose)
- Stomach cramps
- Nausea

Moderate
- Hives

Severe
- Breathing issues
- Swelling of lips, tongue, throat or face

Seek medical attention immediately if you notice any of the moderate to severe side effects or any other adverse side effects.

5. Angiotensin-Converting Enzyme (ACE) Inhibitors.

What are Angiotensin-converting enzyme inhibitors?

Ace inhibitors relax the blood vessels by preventing angiotensin from actually forming. This then widens the blood vessels and makes it easier for the blood to flow.

What are the possible side effects of ACE inhibitors?

Mild
- Dry cough
- Headache

Moderate
- Hives
- Irregular heartbeat
- Dizziness

Severe

- Trouble breathing
- Swelling of throat, tongue, lips or face

6. Beta Blockers

What are beta blockers?

Beta blockers (or beta-adrenergic blocking agents) work to block the effects of adrenaline (epinephrine) and thus help your heart to beat less force and at a slower pace, which in turn helps open up the blood pressures to improve the blood flow thus helping to regulate your blood pressure.

What are the possible side effects of beta blockers?

Mild
- Shortness of breath
- Sleeping issues
- Mild depression

Moderate
- Coldness in the extremities (hands, feet)
- Fatigue
- Weight gain

Severe
- Rapid heartbeat
- Asthma-like attacks

If you experience any of the severe symptoms or any other unusual symptoms, you should seek immediate medical attention.

7. Calcium Channel Blockers

What are calcium channel blockers?

Calcium channel blockers prevent calcium from entering the blood vessel and heart muscle cells which causes them to relax thus making it easier for the heart to pump blood which eases the pressure on the blood vessels and in turn helps regulate blood pressure.

What are the possible side effects of calcium channel blockers?

Mild
- Constipation
- Drowsiness
- Nausea

Moderate
- Headache
- Dizziness
- Flushing
- Rash

Severe
- Heart palpitations
- Swelling in the lower legs and feet

As with any medication, you should seek immediate medical attention if you start to experience any of the severe side effects, as well as any other adverse reactions

8. Central-Acting Agents

What are central-acting agents?
Central-acting agents aid in that they prevent your brain from sending signals to your central nervous system which causes your heart rate to speed up and your blood vessels to narrow. T

This then prevents your heart from pumping so hard so it is now easier for your blood to flow through your blood vessels which ultimately lowers your blood pressure.

What are the possible side effects of central-acting agents?

Mild
- Fever
- Dry mouth
- Fatigue

Moderate
- Dizziness
- Constipation

Severe
- Abnormally slow heart rate

If you notice any of these severe side effects or experience any other adverse reactions seek medical care immediately.

9. Diuretics

What are Diuretics?
Diuretics are essentially water pills. They work to remove any excess sodium and water from your body. This helps to lower the fluid that is flows to your blood vessels thus reducing the

pressure. There are many types of diuretics available and your doctor will recommend the one that works well for you. The following are the different types of diuretics that are available to help lower your blood pressure.

Thiazide diuretics: These are usually recommended as a first line of treatment for those who are suffering from hypertension. They are usually prescribed with at least one other medication.

Loop diuretics: These are most often prescribed for those who have kidney issues and heart conditions or some type of edema (swelling) in addition to blood pressure issues.

Quinazoline diuretics: These are similar to thiazide diuretics but are used for those who have kidney issues or for those who have not had success with other types of diuretics.

For those who have issues with potassium, such as low potassium levels, your doctor may prescribe a potassium-sparing diuretic.

Possible Side Effects of Diuretics

Mild
- Stomach pains
- Sensitivity to light (skin)
- Nausea
- Decreased appetite

Moderate
- Hives
- Confusion

- Dry mouth
- Numbness or tingling in extremities (hands and feet)
- Irregular heartbeat

Severe
- Swelling of throat, face, lips or tongue
- Difficulty breathing

Of course you need to seek medical attention immediately if you have any of the moderate to severe side effects or any other adverse effects to these or any other medications.

10. Renin Inhibitors

What are renin inhibitors?
Renin inhibitors work to block renin, thus relaxing the blood vessels which make it easier for the blood to flow, thus lowering blood pressure.

What are the possible side effects of renin inhibitors?

Mild
- Stuffy nose
- Dizziness

Moderate
- Persistent headache
- Hives

Severe
- Breathing difficulties
- Swelling of the face, lips, throat or tongue

Contact your physician and seek immediate help if you suffer from any of the moderate to severe side effects or experience any other adverse effects from taking renin inhibitors.

11. Vasodilators

What are vasodilators?

Vasodilators work to dilate (or open) the blood vessels by preventing the muscles in the arteries and veins to tighten and thus narrow making your blood flow easier so your heart will not have to work as hard.

What are the possible side effects of vasodilators?

Mild
- Joint pain
- Flushed face
- Nausea

Moderate
- Vomiting
- Dizziness
- Headache

Severe
- Heart palpitations
- Edema (fluid retention)
- Chest pain

As with any of the medications above, you should contact your physician and seek immediate medical help if you experience any of the moderate to severe side effects of this medication, as well as any other adverse effects.

Managing Your Blood Pressure with Vitamins and Supplements

In some cases, there are vitamins and supplements that you can take either in conjunction with your prescription medications that can help regulate and lower your blood pressure. In some cases, you may be able to take these instead of prescriptions. However, before taking any vitamins, supplements or other over-the counter medication or remedy, you should discuss your options in detail with your physician. Never take anything without proper medical advice and consent. Always discuss any and all medications, supplements, etc you are taking with your physician as you do not know if how they will interact with other medications you may be taken or cause adverse effects.

The following is a list of vitamins and other supplements that might help to lower your blood pressure. Again be sure to talk to your physician before adding any of these supplements to your daily regime.

Vitamin D

Research has indicated that there is a direct link between high blood pressure and vitamin D. Those who have higher levels of vitamin D are less likely to develop hypertension and overall have better blood pressure levels. However, as you can overdose on any vitamin, it is recommended that you take less than 10,000 IU of Vitamin D per day. You should discuss what amount of Vitamin D would be beneficial for you with your physician. Vitamin D should not be taken in place of your prescribed medications, but rather in conjunction.

Coenzyme Q10 (CoQ10)

Coenzyme Q10 is powerful antioxidant that is naturally found in almost every cell in our bodies that helps convert our food into energy. Studies have revealed that taking CoQ10 can help lower diastolic blood pressure by as much as 10 mmHg and diastolic blood pressure by as much as 17 mm Hg without any substantial or noticeable side effects.

Magnesium

Magnesium has been proven to help lower blood pressure. It can prevent your heart muscles from spams, prevent and dissolve blood clots, and dilate blood vessels to reduce and regulate hypertension. Magnesium may be taken as a supplement (usually 500 mg daily) or found in certain foods that may be added to your diet. Foods that contain significant amounts of magnesium include almonds, avocado, green leafy vegetables and beans and legumes. You should discuss adding magnesium to your diet with your physician. Magnesium deficiencies are believed to be one of the contributors to high blood pressure.

Vitamin E

Vitamin E has been proven to reduce both diastolic and systolic blood pressure as well as aid in regulating the heart rate. Vitamin E affects the production of nitric oxide, which aids in relaxing the smooth muscles of the arteries, thus putting less pressure on the vein and blood vessels. However, those who are taking a prescribed dose of beta blockers should not take a large amount of Vitamin E as it may interfere with the absorption of the beta blockers. As always, talk to your physician before adding any vitamins or supplements to your diet.

Conclusion

Whether you are prescribed medication by your doctor, or if you are taking any of the above vitamins or supplements (or anything else suggested by your primary care physician), you need to ensure that you follow the directions given to you and stop taking the medication and/or contact your physician if you experience any adverse reactions. If you experience any of the severe side effects that were discussed early in this chapter (hives, shortness of breath, heart palpitations, etc) you need to seek immediate medical care.

Every case is different and certain medications might not work for you so you need to keep your regularly scheduled appointments with your physician, as well as keep a record of your blood pressure. Only your doctor can determine if you can change medications if one isn't working for you. This also applies to ending medications. If your doctor has determined that your blood pressure is under control, he/she may tell you to stop taking your medication. Then they will monitor your blood pressure rate for a specified period of time to decide if you continue to go without medication. If they determine that you were making more progress with the prescribed medication, they may advise you to restart your dosage.

As with any medication, you should never start or stop taking your blood pressure medication, as well as increase or decrease your dosage without first talking to your physician. Never take any medication that has not been prescribed for you by your personal doctor. Read and follow all directions carefully.

Medication, prescription or otherwise, is a serious matter that should not be taken lightly. If you disagree with what your physician is telling you, it won't hurt to get a second opinion, but never make a decision regarding your medication on your own. It could literally mean the difference between life and death.

While medication is normally the best course to regulate blood pressure, there are other things you can do to help control your hypertension. In the next chapter we shall discuss how to manage low blood pressure (hypotension) and in Chapter 4 and the remaining chapters of this eBooks we shall discuss ways you can manage your blood pressure without medication (or in addition to your medication) from diet to medication to helpful tips for everyday life.

CHAPTER THREE

Managing Low Blood Pressure

While most people think that low blood pressure is something to strive for (rather than high blood pressure), low blood pressure can be cause for concern. As discussed in the first chapter it can be an indicator of a more serious illness from diabetes to heart issues. It might also be an indicator of pregnancy in women. If you are suffering from any of the symptoms of hypotension/low blood pressure that were discussed in Chapter 1, you should see your physician. These include (but are not limited to) dizziness, fatigue, excessive thirst, rapid heartbeat, blurred vision, etc.

There are many ways to treat low blood pressure without medication. It is much easier to manage than high blood pressure, in most instances. However, this does not mean that you should take it lightly. You need to regulate your blood pressure before it becomes a serious health concern.

In the following section we shall discuss some ways you can help raise your blood pressure. Again, we can't stress enough how important it is that you should discuss your individual situation with your doctor before making an drastic changes or implementing any new changes into your diet or lifestyle such as over the counter medications or supplements.

Drink More Water

Water is so beneficial for your health. We simply cannot stress this enough. However, it is especially beneficial to increase your water intake if you are suffering from low blood pressure. One of the causes of low blood pressure is dehydration. Drinking more water will not only hydrate your body but it will increase your blood volume thus helping to raise your blood pressure.

Wear Compression Stockings

Compression stockings have been proven to help increase the blood flow in the legs, which can greatly help increase your blood pressure. However, it is important to make sure that you are getting the proper type and brand of compression stockings. You can discuss this with your physician and you can also go to a medical supply store to be fitted properly for compression stockings.

Avoid Alcohol

Alcohol has proven to be a hindrance to both high and low blood pressure as well as overall circulatory system and heart health. Over time it destroys the nerves that would aid in constricting the blood vessels. It also increases the excretion of liquid and reduces the overall performance of the heart. Whether you have been diagnosed with hypertension or hypotension, you should either greatly reduce your alcohol intake or eliminate alcohol altogether to regulate your blood pressure.

Increase Your Salt Intake

While those with high blood pressure should greatly cut back on sodium, the opposite is true for those who suffer from low blood pressure. Increasing your sodium level will increase the liquids in the body which will in turn increase your blood pressure. It is recommended that those with hypotension increase their salt intake primarily in the morning.

This being said, those with other complications such as heart issues or those women who are pregnant or nursing should stick to a low-sodium diet. You should definitely discuss your particular situation with your doctor before increasing your salt intake.

Additional Tips to Help Raise Low Blood Pressure

1. When standing up from lying or sitting down, be sure not to get up to quickly. This can cause a drop in your blood pressure. In order to increase your circulation massage your feet or ankles (if possible) before getting up, or simply pump your feet a few times. When you first awaken in the morning, sit on the edge of your bed for a few minutes before standing up.

2. Avoid lifting heavy objects as much as possible. Ask for assistance.

3. Eat smaller meals throughout the day and drink a glass of water once an hour.

4. Avoid carbohydrates and eat more green leafy vegetables.

5. Avoid prolonged exposure to heat (i.e.: hot showers, saunas, hot tubs overexposure to humidity/sun, etc). If you have to be exposed to higher temperatures or humidity, drink plenty of water and stop to rest. Do not overexert yourself.

6. Exercise regularly to increase your circulation.

7. Increase your Vitamin B12 consumption. Foods such as fish and dairy can help raise your Vitamin B12 levels which in turn will help raise your blood pressure. You can also ask your physician if taking a Vitamin B12 supplement will benefit your specific condition.

Conclusion

As previously stated, low blood pressure can be caused by several factors such as an underlying health condition or as a side effect of certain medications. You need to disclose all of your information regarding your health and any medications you may be taking to your physician, as well as your full medical history. Truthfully answer any questions your physician may have as this will help them to determine what course of treatment may be best for you.

While low blood pressure is often short-term and usually easier to control then high blood pressure, it may be an indicator of a more serious condition, so low blood pressure should not be taken lightly.

In the next chapter we shall discuss ways to regulate your blood pressure without medication through changes in diet as well as exercise.

CHAPTER FOUR

How to Manage Blood Pressure without Medication

Now that we have taken a look at the various medications that can be used to treat high blood pressure, it is time to examine ways to regulate your blood pressure without medication. Medication can be beneficial, and at times life-saving, but you don't want to have to rely on medications for the rest of your life, as many of them have long-term side effects, not to mention they can be quite costly. There are plenty of ways to lower or regulate your blood pressure rate without taking medication. Studies have indicated that over 85% of people with blood pressure issues can learn to control their blood pressure without the use of medication.

In this chapter we shall take a look at factors such as diet, exercise and vitamins and supplements that can help control your blood pressure. Simple changes can make a big difference in regulating your blood pressure, as well as your overall health.

Diet

If you look online or in health journals, there are plenty of diets that are designed to help you both control your blood pressure and lose weight. In this section, we shall take a look at some of the major food groups as well as some different diet plans that you can use to help regulate your blood pressure.

Obviously, making healthier choices can increase your overall health. As a general rule you should aim for a diet that is rich in the following:

- Vegetables
- Fruit
- Grains
- Dairy
- Legumes
- Lean Meats
- Seafood

We shall discuss these more in depth in this section as well as give you some helpful tips for alternative diets that you can follow that are specifically geared for controlling blood pressure.

DASH Diet

If you have been diagnosed with high blood pressure, your doctor may recommend that you follow the Dash Diet. You can check out their website for more detailed information, but we will give you a breakdown of the essentials. The DASH Diet has been rated as the most effective diet for treating hypertension for the past six years, as well as for weight loss, diabetes, osteoporosis, and lowering cholesterol as well as overall heart health.

The DASH (Dietary Approaches to Stop Hypertension) Diet focuses on regulating portion size while still being able to eat a variety of foods that contain the proper amount of nutrients. It also helps you greatly lower your sodium intake. The DASH Diet contains a large number of foods that are rich in calcium, potassium and magnesium, which have been proven to help reduce blood pressure levels.

By following the DASH Diet, you may be able to lower your blood pressure in just as a matter of weeks. If you adhere strictly to the DASH Diet, you may be able to reduce your systolic blood pressure by up to 14 points.

There are 2 version of the DASH Diet available, according to the amount of sodium. We will discuss how lowering sodium can greatly lower your blood pressure levels in depth in Chapter 4. You should never begin any type of self-treatment or diet for hypertension without first discussing it with your doctor. Your doctor will also be able to determine how much what sodium level is best for your health.

For the purposes of this eBook, we shall base the following information for the DASH Diet for the average caloric consumption of 2,000 calories a day. It is important that you incorporate the various food groups into your daily regimen and follow the diet so you can achieve optimum results in lowering and controlling your blood pressure.

Dairy (2-3 servings daily)

Dairy products such as milk, cheese and yogurt are ideal sources of calcium, protein and Vitamin D. There has been much debate as to whether it is healthier to eat full vs. low or no fat. When trying to lower your blood pressure, it is recommended that you consume dairy that is lower in fat. While full fat is not as bad as some say it is, it is better for those who are trying to reduce their blood pressure to consume less fat.

The following items are examples of dairy products that are recommended for the DASH Diet:

- Skim or 1 percent milk
- Low fat greek or regular yogurt
- Part-skim cheeses

Regular cheeses and even some reduced-fat cheeses tend to be high in sodium. Also if you cannot digest dairy, it you can opt for lactose-free milk.

Lean Meats, Poultry and Seafood (n more than 6 servings per day)

Lean meats and poultry are an excellent source of B vitamins, zinc, and iron and of course, protein. Seafood such as shellfish and fish that are low in mercury are rich in minerals, vitamins, and protein and omega-3 fatty acids. It is recommended that you limit your seafood servings to two servings per week as some fish can be higher in sodium. Fish such as tuna, herring and salmon are known to be very high in Omega-3 fatty acids and have been proven to help reduce cholesterol

You should make sure that any meat, poultry and seafood that you consume are cleaned properly and thoroughly cooked. You should remove the skin and trim away any fat from poultry and lean meats. It is recommended that you should avoid frying and stick to broiling, grilling, baking or roasting instead.

Vegetables (4-5 servings daily)

Vegetables are rich in many nutrients including B Vitamins, Vitamins A and C, folic acids, fiber, zinc, iron, magnesium and potassium. Green leafy vegetables are an excellent source of nutrients. You don't have to limit vegetables to just a "side dish" during your evening meal. They make an excellent snack or even a full meal, when prepared as a casserole or stir fry. Below are examples of some of the vegetables that are including in the DASH Diet:

- Broccoli
- Carrots
- Sweet Potatoes
- Kale
- Spinach
- Collard Greens
- Turnips
- Green Beans
- Brussel Sprouts

Of course, fresh vegetables are best, but frozen vegetables are good as well. You should avoid canned vegetables are often high in sodium. If you do purchase frozen or canned vegetables, check the sodium levels before you make your selection.

Fruit (4- 5 servings per day)

Fruit is also full of magnesium, potassium, fiber and vitamins and are generally very low in fat. You can snack on fruit and use it as a side dish in a meal or in a salad. You can also add fruit to yogurt along with granola for a tasty and nutritious snack. You can also make smoothies or add fruit to multigrain and healthy cereals or oatmeal. Both fruits and veggies are extremely versatile so you have hundreds of options and no excuses not to add them to your daily diet.

The following fruits are a good source of nutrition and are especially good for lowering and regulating your blood pressure:

- Apples
- Oranges
- Pears
- Plums
- Apricots
- Pineapple
- Mango
- Bananas
- Berries
- Grapes
- Avocado
- Tomato
- Lemon
- Cantaloupe

- Grapefruit
- Prunes

Grains (6-8 daily servings)

Grains contain a high amount of nutrients including fiber, folate, riboflavin, iron, selenium and magnesium and niacin. Of course, with the awareness of celiac disease and those who have gluten and wheat intolerances, there is much debate about grains. But for those who have sensitivity issues, there are plenty of grains that are gluten free.

Whole grains are richer in fiber than refined grains so it is better to opt for whole grain bread as opposed to white bread, or white rice as opposed to brown rice. Grains are also low in fat. Grains that are beneficial to regulating blood pressure include the following:

- Brown rice
- Whole wheat pasta
- Multi grain bread
- Oats
- Multi grain cereals
- Granola
- Quinoa
- Millet
- Barley
- Buckwheat

Oils & Fats (2- 3 servings a day)

Fats get a bad rap, but they are healthy fats are actually good for you as they help our bodies absorb vitamins while also strengthening our immune systems. However, we need to make sure that we are consuming only healthy fats. Too much fat can increase our risks of obesity, heart disease and diabetes. On the DASH Diet, you should have have 2-3 servings of healthy fats a day. Make sure that you are reading labels to see the recommended serving size per portion. You should avoid saturated and Trans fats as much as possible. Examples of healthy fats include the following:

- Grass-fed butter
- Salad dressings
- Olive Oil
- Grapeseed Oil
- Avocado Oil
- Coconut OIl
- Palm Oil

Seeds, Nuts & Legumes/bean (4-5 servings per week)

Nuts, seeds, and legumes are an excellent source of protein, fiber, potatoes and magnesium, as well as phytochemicals. They should only be consumed four to five times a week due to their high caloric content. The following are recommended for the DASH Diet:

- Almonds
- Walnuts
- Peanuts
- Cashews
- Kidney beans
- Black beans
- Black-eyed peas

- Lentils
- Sunflower seeds
- Flax seeds
- Chia seeds
- Tofu
- Tempah

Other factors of the DASH Diet including eliminated or greatly reducing sugar intake, and alcohol and caffeine as well, you should avoid refined sugars as much as possible and rely on fruit as your main source of sugar. Alcohol and caffeine can significantly raise your blood pressure so you should either completely eliminate them from your diet, or greatly reduce your overall intake.

In addition to the DASH diet, there are several foods that are especially beneficial to reducing and regulating blood pressure. These include the following:

- Tilapia
- Kiwi
- Pork Tenderloin
- White beans
- Peaches
- Nectarines
- Red pepper
- Beets
- Garlic
- Turmeric
- Green teas and green coffees

- Skim milk
- Dark chocolate
- Soybeans
- Mushrooms
- Lima beans

Potassium has been shown to significantly reduce blood pressure. Potassium naturally counteracts the negative effects of sodium. Of course, this does not mean that by increasing your calcium intake you can thus increase your sodium intake. In Chapter 5 we shall discuss in depth how sodium affects your blood pressure health.

Exercise

Exercise is beneficial for our bodies for so many reasons, but it can also help significantly lower blood pressure. Physical activity strengthens our hearts which then enables our hearts to pump blood with much less effort than if we do not exercise. As the burden of working harder to pump blood decreases so does the pressure on the arteries which then lowers our blood pressure.

Physical activity greatly lowers our systolic blood pressure level by as much as 9 mm HG, which is just as effective, if not more so, than most blood pressure medications. A great number of people over the years have completely eliminated the need for medication simply by incorporating physical exercise into their daily routine.

Of course, this will not happen instantaneously. You need to exercise consistently for about two or three months to notice a positive impact on your blood pressure. And of course you have to keep it up. It will not be beneficial if you start out with a great exercise program and significantly lower your blood pressure only to stop exercising and watch as it increases again. Consistency is the key...with diet and exercise as well.

How much exercise is beneficial in lowering blood pressure?

To regulate your blood pressure it is recommended that you should get at least 150 minutes of moderate exercise a week, or 75 minutes of intense activity. The best recommendation is 30 minutes a day at least 4 days a week. This does not mean that you should not exercise at all on your "off days." Simply taking a brisk ten minute walk is beneficial for both your heart health and your blood pressure.

For those who have an exceptionally busy day, you can break up your thirty minutes of physical activity into 2 fifteen minutes or 3 ten minutes bursts of high impact activity. Also, if you have an office job or another job where you are off your feet most of the day, you should take at least 5 minutes and hour and take a quick walk or at least stand up and stretch. Spending too much time sedentary can contribute to high blood pressure. And as we have stated many times, stress also contributes to high blood pressure. Exercise greatly reduces anxiety so at the same time it can help lower your blood pressure. It's a win-win situation. Add in bonus points for those who are trying to lose weight or get into better overall physical physique.

What type of exercise is beneficial to lowering and regulating blood pressure?

Any type of physical and aerobic activity can help control your blood pressure. You don't necessarily have to go out and join a gym. Kudos to you if you chose to do so, but you can easily exercise in the privacy of your own home. Below are just some suggestions for physical activity

- Walking
- Jogging
- Treadmill
- Dancing
- Aerobics classes
- Spinning classes
- Zumba
- Jazzercise
- Team sports (softball, football, soccer, basketball, etc)
- Tennis
- Skiing
- Swimming
- Power-walking
- Stair climbing
- Bicycling
- Running

Even activities such as housework can be considered physical activity: gardening, raking leaves, mowing the lawn and other such yard work, scrubbing floors, vacuuming, etc are all physical activities. If you don't want to join a gym, there are plenty of workout videos you can purchase in the store or on

Amazon or Ebay. And there are hundreds of exercise videos on sites such as Youtube. And if you aren't a fan of typical aerobics, you can easily put on your favorite music and dance around your home. You don't have to be super-coordinated or an Olympic athlete to exercise. It's as simple as getting off your couch and going for a brisk walk around the block.

You can also take "shortcuts" as well. Take the stairs instead of the elevator or escalator. Park a little farther back at the store so you have a longer walk. Walk to work or for errands if possible. Every little bit of physical activity adds us.

There are plenty of apps for your smartphone or tablet that you can use to help keep track of your exercise..And your diet as well, LoseIt and MyFitnessPal are two of the most popular apps. And for those who are really serious about their diet and exercise routine, you could always purchase a FitBit!

Of course, it goes without being said, that you should consult your physician before undertaking any type of physical activity. Your health and safety are your first concern. Your doctor can recommend what type of exercise is best for you.

Conclusion

Diet and exercise are crucial for a long and healthy life, regardless of any underlying medical issues. However, for those who have been diagnosed with any medication condition, a proper diet and physical exercise are critical to maintaining good health. Before you make any diet, exercise or any other lifestyle changes you need to talk to your primary care physician or specialist. Simple changes in your diet, ,as well as the proper amount of exercises (based on your individual circumstances) can greatly improve your blood pressure level, and your overall health.

In the following chapter, we shall discuss how meditation and yoga can help naturally control your blood pressure. These forms of relaxation therapy have been proven to have a significant effect in blood pressure regulation.

CHAPTER FIVE

Using Meditation and/or Yoga to help regulate your blood pressure

Both yoga and meditation have been proven to be extremely beneficial in lowering and regulating blood pressure in combination with diets such as the DASH diet and an exercise regime. In the following chapter we shall discuss how these and other relaxation exercises can help regulate your blood pressure.

For those who are overly concerned about strenuous physical activity or those who might have other health issues such a heart condition in addition to high blood pressure, yoga and/or meditation might extremely beneficial in helping to lower blood pressure levels without putting too much physical stress on the body. And either way, both are extremely relaxing and fairly easy to do, so it's a win/win situation.

You don't need to join a gym or pay for private yoga classes. You can look for online courses or information. And we will give you a simplified breakdown of both, as well as how they can be beneficial in controlling your blood pressure.

Meditation

Another way to lower and regulate your blood pressure is through meditation. Meditation is a relaxing and easy way to put your mind at ease. There are many health benefits with meditation. You could take a class or practice in the privacy of your own home. In this chapter, we shall discuss how meditation can help regulate your blood pressure and give you a brief tutorial on how to practice mediation, as well as how to incorporate mindfulness into your everyday life.

How exactly does meditation help lower blood pressure?

One of the benefits of meditation is that it practices controlled breathing, which increases the nitric oxide production in our bodies. This will in turn help open the blood vessels, thus causing less pressure and helping to regulate our blood pressure levels.

Meditation alone cannot lower your blood pressure. You should practice meditation along with exercise and diet in order to regulate your blood pressure. Studies have indicated that those who regularly practice meditation in conjunction with diet and exercise can drastically lower their blood pressure without the use of medication.

Mindfulness Meditation

There are many different types of meditation, but perhaps the most common type is mindfulness meditation. But what exactly is mindfulness meditation?

Mindfulness meditation is simply the process of focusing your attention on both the internal and external events of the moment at hand. It takes your focus off of the events that may have caused you anxiety in the past as well as future events that might be causing you additional, and often unnecessary stress, which can greatly affect your blood pressure. It will help you to focus solely on the present and help you remain calm and be able to enjoy the moment at hand.

Below is a simple guide on how to practice mindfulness meditation. We shall also give you some ideas on how to incorporate mindfulness into your daily life to help eliminate stress and regulate your blood pressure.

Guide to Practicing Mindfulness Meditation

1. Choose a time and place

You should find a time of the day, as well as a location, where you can be free from all distraction, Maybe a quiet corner in your home office, or bedroom, Or perhaps a quiet place outdoors...in your backyard or even in the woods or the on the beach. Whatever area works best for you...one in which you will feel safe at completely at ease. You can meditate first thing in the morning to set the tone for your day, or before you go to sleep at night, to help you relax. That is the beauty of mindfulness meditation, it is very private and personal and you can easily adjust it to fit your own personal needs and schedule.

2. Relax, clear your mind and take several deep breaths.

Position yourself so that you are completely comfortable. Rid yourself of all distractions. You can sit or kneel or choose whichever position works best for you. Those are no set position for mindfulness meditation. Next take several deep relaxing breaths (slow breaths so you don't pass out) and empty your mind. Of course, emptying your mind will not be an easy task, but you will get better over time.

3. Focus on the moment at hand

What are you feeling at this *exact moment?* What do you see? Smell? Hear? What is going through your mind. Let the present moment completely wash over you. Surrender yourself to the *here and now.*

Again, this may take practice. But the more you practice, the easier it will become. You will find yourself becoming more and more relaxed and you will find it easier to focus on the task at hand.

How to incorporate mindfulness into your everyday life

You might be thinking "Great, sure mindfulness meditation can help me calm down at night before I go to bed or in the morning, but that's only short-term. How can I use it do help keep me calm during the day.?"

That is the beauty of mindfulness. You can practice it wherever you want, whenever you want. You don't have to be sitting lotus style on the beach or in a room with candlelight. You can practice mindfulness meditation anytime of the day or night.

You can start with practicing mindfulness from the very second you open your eyes. Instead of reaching for your phone to check your Facebook or Twitter account, take a few moments to center yourself and focus on the moment. Start your day off in the present and it will help you to stay focused during the day.

You can practice while you are taking your shower, or making your breakfast, or during your commute to work. Or take a few minutes on your lunch break. Whatever works best for you. The more time you take to practice mindfulness, the easier it will become for you to stay focused on the moment. You will stop fretting over the past and worrying about the future. As you start to feel more at peace, your blood pressure levels will start to regulate.

Again, this will not happen overnight. If you are taking medication, you may have to continue to do so until your doctor tells you otherwise. But through the power of meditation, a change in your diet and exercise, you will be able to greatly lower your blood pressure rate and live a healthier lifestyle.

How Yoga Can Help Regulate Your Blood Pressure

Yoga is the combination of spiritual, physical and mental disciplines that encompasses low impact physical activity (mainly stretching), meditation and controlled breathing to help you relax and also achieve a higher form of consciousness. Studies have indicated that the calming effects of yoga can have a positive effect in lowering blood pressure.

As some people who have been diagnosed with hypertension have also been diagnosed with heart problems, aerobic and/or strenuous exercise is not always recommended. Yoga, unlike intense physical exercise does not put additional stress on the cardiovascular system. This in turns increases the both the blood pressure and heart rate.

Yoga, however, is not tremendous and does not put additional physical stress on the body. Instead, it is relaxing. Yoga poses can help the body to find a focus between the physical, spiritual and mental realms, therefore lowering the level of stress and lowering blood pressure. In fact, there are certain yoga positions that have been specially classified as "health health" or cardiovascular yoga, as these positions put less pressure on the heart which can in turn help control your blood pressure.

Recommended Yoga Poses to Help Lower Blood Pressure

Of course, before you attempt to undertake yoga, you should discuss this with your physician. And if possible, do not attempt any of these positions on your own, at least the first few times. Find a yoga class specifically designed for cardiovascular yoga or practice with a trusted friend or family member. The following yoga positions are those that have have been proven to be most effective for helping to lower blood pressure, but are not to be taken lightly or attempted without proper training.

There are actually quite a few yoga poses for cardiovascular yoga that will help regulate blood pressure, but for purposes of this eBook we will give you the top 5 recommended poses. You can find tutorial videos online on sites such as YouTube and you can also find the other recommended sites as well (see the reference section at the end of the eBook for some other resources on cardiovascular yoga positions)

1. Bridge Pose (Setu Bandha Sarvangasana)

1. Lie on your back with your feet on the floor and your knees bent. You can put a pillow underneath your neck and or back to prevent injury.

2. Extend your arms next to your body with your palms facing down.

3. Press your arms and feet firmly on the ground and slowly exhale as you raise your hips upward.

4. Slowly pull your tailbone toward the pelvic bone, keeping your bottom off the floor. Do not flex your buttocks.

5. Slowly roll your shoulders back till they are underneath you. Clasp your hands together and raise your arms beneath your pelvis along the floor. Then straighten them as much as you can while pressing your forearms onto the floor, keeping your knuckles facing your heel.

6. Do not roll onto your feet or let your knees drop. Evenly distribute your weight and putt your tailbone toward the back of your needs while keeping your feet and thighs parallel.

2. Corpse Pose (Savasana)

1. Lie flat on your back on the floor, Keep your arms and legs straight (arms at your sides).

2. Place your hands about 6 inches from your body, palms facing upward,

3. Relax your feet.

4. Close your eyes.

5. Breathe regularly and let your body feel heavy to the ground,

6. Consciously relax every single part of your body including your organs, staring from your toes and working your way to the top of your head.

7. Once you feel relaxed, let a sense of complete inner peace and calm take over. Since your body, mind and soul.

8. Remain in this position for up to 30 minutes with no interruptions.

3. Downward Facing Dog (Adho Mukha Shvanasana)

1. Get down on your hands and knees.

2. Align yourself so that your wrists are directly underneath your shoulders and your knees are directly underneath your hips. Your wrists should be parallel to the top edge of your yoga mat, with your middle fingers point directly to the edge.

3. Relax your upper back,

4. Stretch your elbow.

5. Spread your fingers as wide as you can while pressing firmly on your palms and knuckles, making sure to evenly distribute your weight across your hands.

6. Tuck your toe and slowly raise your knees and pelvis toward the ceiling, drawing your backside toward the wall. Slowly straighten your legs without locking your knees in place. Your body should be in the shape of an "A." Keep your body extended, do not place.

7. Lifting your pelvis slowly press away from the floor. As your spine is lengthening, lift your buttocks toward the ceiling. Then press your weight down through the palms of your hands and your heels.

8. Press your index fingers firmly on the floor as you lift the muscles of your arms to the tops of your shoulders while drawing your shoulder blades toward your upper back ribs and toward your buttocks.

9. Then rotate your arms so the crease of your elbows faces your thumbs and draw your chest toward your thighs.

10. Rotate your thighs inward and sink your heels to the floor. Then align your upper arms with your ears, relaxed, but not dangling, your head.

4. Hero Pose (Virasana)

1. Kneel on the floor placing a pillow or folded blanket underneath your feet, knees and shins. Keep your hips perpendicular to the floor. Your inner thighs should be touching.

2. Spread your feet so they are just a little bit wider than your hips. Keep the tops of your feet lat and your toes should be facing each other as you press evenly across the tops of your feet.

3. Exhale as you lean your torso slightly forward while sitting your hips halfway back. Reach back with your thighs drawn in to your calf muscles toward your heel rounding your back ever-so-slightly.

4. Place your body on your feet, in a sitting posting so your weight is evenly distributed. Make sure your shins and heels are next to your upper thighs and hips; your feet should be directly in line with your shins, but do not lean your feet inward.

5. Slightly turn your thighs in while pressing down on them with your hands.

6. Sit up straight, bringing your shoulder blades toward your back ribs firmly. Drop your shoulders away from your ears, lengthen your tailbone toward the floor and drop your shoulders away from your ears. Then place your hands on your upper thighs, palms facing downward.

5. Legs Up On The Wall Pose (Viparita Karani)

1. Sit with the left side of your body against a sturdy wall. If you are using a pillow or other such prop for support, your lower back should be resting against that (of course the pillow, etc should be lying flat against the wall)

2. Slowly and gently turn your entire body to the left and place your legs on the wall, using your hands to keep your balance.

3. Slowly and carefully lower your back to the floor.

4. Lie down, resting your shoulders and head comfortably on the floor.

5. Shifting your weight from side to side, slide your buttocks as close as you can to the wall.

6. Keep your arms relaxed at your side, keeping your palms facing upward.

7. Relax your thighs and pelvis and close your eyes.

8. Focus on relaxed breathing and awareness for up to ten minutes.

Again, do not attempt any of these cardiovascular yoga poses without first consulting your doctor. You need to make sure that you are physically able to sustain these positions and you also don't want to attempt any of these positions without assistance, at least the first few times until you have perfected them.

As you can see, yoga benefits the entire cardiovascular system starting with the blood flow to improve circulation. It also helps rejuvenate your blood cells and helps to keep the blood vessels elastic by stretching the walls of the blood vessels. Yoga lao helps fresh nutrients and oxygen flow to the necessary organs thus improving circulation. This can help regulate your blood pressure as well as elevate your mood and improve your sleeping habits, which in turn have a positive effect on your blood pressure health.

Conclusion

When properly practiced on a regular basis, both yoga and meditation can help lower and control your blood pressure. While physical exercise may benefit some, yoga and meditation may work better for others. All it takes is discipline and practice.

Whether you are engaging in some type of cardiovascular exercise or relaxation therapy such as yoga, controlled breathing or meditation (or all of the above), you need to make it a part of your daily routine. Set aside time for your daily reference and make it a critical part of your day, as much as you would eating or personal hygiene. Taking care of your physical and mental health can have a great effect on reducing and regulating your blood pressure.

There are plenty of online resources and videos available to assist you with both yoga and meditation. You can also find local classes and groups for both. It is always a good idea to find a support group, at least a friend, to practice with you and it will give you extra motivation. There are even apps available for your smartphone or tablet to assist you with guided meditation and relaxation exercises. Thanks to technology, there is an unlimited amount of resources available on both meditation and yoga right at your fingertips.

In the next chapter we shall offer you some additional tips on how to regulate your blood pressure from subtle changes in diet such as cutting back on caffeine to lifestyle changes such as time management. With or without prescription medication, these small changes can have a huge impact on your blood pressure as well as your overall health.

CHAPTER SIX

Tips to Control your Blood Pressure

In addition to what we medication, diet and exercise (including yoga and meditation) there are other simple lifestyle changes you can do to help regulate your blood pressure. We shall discuss these in this chapter and give you some advice in how to lower your blood pressure and maintain a healthy level.

1. Drink Green Tea

Green tea contains a high level of polyphenol antioxidants that are beneficial in lowering blood pressure. Included in these are flavonoids, which contain catechins, which have are beneficial in fighting and preventing many types of illnesses. Green tea also contains less caffeine than other teas, this helping to ease levels of anxiety, which can also affect your blood pressure. Simply switching from coffee to green tea can greatly lower your blood pressure. Studies have shown that those who drink at least four cups of green tea a day significantly lowered their blood pressure levels over time.

For those who do not like to drink tea, green tea is also available in a capsule form. However, you can always add lemon, lime or honey to flavor your tea as well.

2. Switch to Decaf Coffee

For those who cannot simply give up their coffee, switching to decaf coffee is another option. If you really must have caffeine to get you going, you can have one cup of regular coffee, and switch to decaf after that. Also, there are many brand names that sell "half-caff" coffees.

Caffeine raises your blood pressure levels as it tightens your blood vessels. It also intensities stress levels which in turn can raise your blood pressure. Simply by cutting back on your caffeine intake you can lower your blood pressure by 6 mm Hg. Eliminating caffeine altogether can have even a greater effect.

3. Drastically Reduce Salt Intake

This one is the biggie. Sodium is one of the key factors that affect blood pressure. And salt is found in most foods, especially processed foods. If you look at the nutrition information on most food items, you would be shocked at the high levels of sodium that are in the majority of the foods we eat every day.

High levels of salt will not only increase your blood pressure but it can affect your heart and your kidneys as well. Our kidneys remove harmful fluids from our body by passing them into your bladder when it is then removed as urine. If there is too much salt in the bloodstream your kidneys have more difficulty filtering out these harmful fluids. This then puts extra strain on the blood vessels that lead to the kidneys, causing higher blood pressure and also, ultimately, serious damage to your kidneys.

If you simply pay attention when you shop and read the ingredients on the food you are selecting, you can greatly reduce your salt intake. Also, you can do so by not adding extra salt when cooking or to prepared foods. You might find this challenging at first, and you might think that things now have no taste, but you will get used to it in time. There are a great many other spices you can use in meal preparations. Garlic has been proven to reduce blood sugar levels and is also very tasty as well. If you look online, you can find plenty of recipes that are low to no-salt and you will learn creative ways to create find and exciting new recipes for better heart and blood pressure health.

4. Eliminate Stress from Your Life

Okay, so this is easier said than done. Life today is often hectic and stress is a part of everyday life, it seems. While you may not be able to remove yourself completely from the stressors in your life, you can find ways to manage them. The following are some suggestions to help you learn how to manage your stress.

- Time Management: Find ways to more efficiently manage your time. Eliminate things from your schedule that are not absolutely necessary.
- Learn to say no when you feel overburdened.
- Ask for help, rather than try to handle everything on your own terms.

- Take time for yourself. This is not as easy as it seems, but find time for yourself every day. Read a book. Take a hot bath. Go for a walk or a run. Find some downtime for yourself to give yourself a break from the stressors in your everyday life. Listen to relaxing music. Meditate. Practice Yoga. Take time for your hobbies and personal interests.
- Find a support group. Talk to a friend. If needed, seek professional help (individual or group therapy)
- Keep a journal

Conclusion

These few simple tips are ways you can help regulate your blood pressure. They are by no means a miracle cure, but simply extra precautions you can take to help keep your blood pressure under control. Again, you need to follow your doctor's orders and monitor your blood pressure regularly. But simple lifestyle changes such as getting the proper amount of sleep, getting sun and fresh air every day, regular exercise and little changes in diet and lifestyle can greatly benefit your overall health as well as help you regulate your blood pressure.

Conclusion

We hope that you have found the information contained in this eBook on Understand and Controlling Your Blood Pressure to be helpful and informative. Again, we must stress that this is not a diagnostic tool nor should it take the place of any advice your doctor will provide you. Every case is different and with today's advances in both medicine and technology, there is always new research and information, so please discuss your case with your doctor and never assume anything that you read is meant for your specific case.

The purpose of this eBook is to provide you with the information so you can have a basic understanding of blood pressure and how it affects your health. We have provided a brief guide detailing various medications, diet and lifestyle changes and types of treatments that you can use to help regulate your blood pressure. This is meant as a guideline to help you understand your health. We cannot imagine enough how important it is that you discuss your specific case with your doctor and/or specialist

The point of our eBook is to educate and inform, not to make a diagnosis of your specific case. We want to give you peace of mind that you are not alone, that high blood pressure affects a great number of people and that it can be controlled with medication, diet, exercise and basic lifestyle changes. We hope that you have enjoyed our eBook and we thank you for taking the time to read it. We hope that you have gained some insight that can help you lead a happier, healthier lifestyle and that you are cable to help control your blood pressure! We wish you the best of health!

Appendix 1: Glossary of terms:

Blood pressure: pressure of the blood in the circulatory system that is related to the rate and force of the heartbeat as well as the elasticity of the arterial wall.

Diastolic Blood Pressure: the unit of blood pressure that measures the minimum arterial pressure while the ventricles of the heart are relaxed and filled with blood. This is the second (or bottom) number on a blood pressure reading.

Hypertension (high blood pressure): medical condition in which blood pressure is higher than normal and can cause serious health issues such as heart attack or stroke.

Hypotension (low blood pressure): Medical condition, in which the blood pressure is lower than the normal weight, can be an indicator of an underlying medical issue.

Sphygmomanometer: instrument using for measuring blood pressure to determine the systolic and diastolic blood pressure, Consists of a rubber inflatable cuff that is attached to a scale used to measure blood pressure.

Systolic Blood Pressure: the measurement of the maximum arterial pressure during the contraction of the left ventricle of the heart. It is the first (or top) number recorded in blood pressure readings.

Appendix II: References

1. "What is blood pressure? - Blood Pressure UK." 2012. 18 Jul. 2016 <http://www.bloodpressureuk.org/BloodPressureandyou/Thebasics/Bloodpressure>

2. "Low blood pressure: MedlinePlus Medical Encyclopedia." 2016. 18 Jul. 2016 <https://medlineplus.gov/ency/article/007278.htm>

3. "Blood Pressure - Medical News Today." 2014. 18 Jul. 2016 <http://www.medicalnewstoday.com/articles/270644.php>

4. "Understanding Blood Pressure Readings - American Heart Association." 18 Jul. 2016 <http://www.heart.org/HEARTORG/Conditions/HighBloodPressure/AboutHighBloodPressure/Understanding-Blood-Pressure-Readings_UCM_301764_Article.jsp>

5. High Blood Pressure Symptoms - Symptoms of Hypertension." 18 Jul. 2016 <http://www.healthline.com/health/high-blood-pressure-hypertension-symptoms

6. "What are the Symptoms of High Blood Pressure? - American Heart ..." 18 Jul. 2016 <http://www.heart.org/HEARTORG/Conditions/HighBlo

odPressure/SymptomsDiagnosisMonitoringofHighBlood Pressure/What-are-the-Symptoms-of-High-Blood-Pressure_UCM_301871_Article.jsp>

7. "Low blood pressure (hypotension) Symptoms - Mayo Clinic." 2014. 18 Jul. 2016 <http://www.mayoclinic.org/diseases-conditions/low-blood-pressure/basics/symptoms/con-20032298>

8. "Causes of High Blood Pressure: Weight, Diet, Age, and More - WebMD." 2009. 18 Jul. 2016 <http://www.webmd.com/hypertension-high-blood-pressure/guide/blood-pressure-causes>

9. "Causes of High Blood Pressure - NHLBI, NIH." 2014. 18 Jul. 2016 <http://www.nhlbi.nih.gov/health/health-topics/topics/hbp/causes>

10. "Your body - Blood Pressure UK." 2012. 18 Jul. 2016 <http://www.bloodpressureuk.org/BloodPressureandyou/Thebasics/Yourbody>

11. "High blood pressure dangers: Hypertension effects on ... - Mayo Clinic." 2014. 18 Jul. 2016 <http://www.mayoclinic.org/diseases-conditions/high-blood-pressure/in-depth/high-blood-pressure/art-20045868>

12. "Low Blood Pressure Related Diseases & Conditions - MedicineNet." 2012. 19 Jul. 2016 <http://www.medicinenet.com/low_blood_pressure/related-conditions/index.htm>

13. "How You Can Normalize Your Blood Pressure Without Drugs - Mercola." 2011. 30 Jul. 2016 <http://articles.mercola.com/sites/articles/archive/2009/12/15/how-you-can-normalize-your-blood-pressure-without-drugs.aspx>

14. "Diet for High Blood Pressure | Everyday Health." 2016. 30 Jul. 2016 <http://www.everydayhealth.com/high-blood-pressure/guide/diet/>

15. "The DASH Diet for Healthy Weight Loss, Lower Blood Pressure ..." 2003. 30 Jul. 2016 <http://dashdiet.org/>

16. Standard, D. "DASH diet: Healthy eating to lower your blood pressure - Mayo Clinic." 2015. <http://www.mayoclinic.org/healthy-lifestyle/nutrition-and-healthy-eating/in-depth/dash-diet/art-20048456>

17. food/13-power-foods-that-lower-blood-pressure-naturally - Prevention." 2015. 30 Jul. 2016 <http://www.prevention.com/food/13-power-foods-that-lower-blood-pressure-naturally>

18. "11 Foods Scientifically Proven To Lower Your Blood Pressure." 2015. 30 Jul. 2016 <http://www.bodybuilding.com/fun/11-foods-scientifically-proven-to-lower-your-blood-pressure.html>

19. "Blood Pressure : Why potassium helps to lower ... - Blood Pressure UK." 2012. 30 Jul. 2016 <http://www.bloodpressureuk.org/microsites/salt/Home/Whypotassiumhelps>

20. "High blood pressure and exercise - Mayo Clinic." 2014. 30 Jul. 2016 <http://www.mayoclinic.org/diseases-conditions/high-blood-pressure/in-depth/high-blood-pressure/art-20045206>

21. "Choosing blood pressure medications - Mayo Clinic." 2014. 31 Jul. 2016 <http://www.mayoclinic.org/diseases-conditions/high-blood-pressure/in-depth/high-blood-pressure-medication/art-20046280>

22. "Angiotensin II Receptor Blockers (ARBs) for High Blood Pressure." 2007. 31 Jul. 2016 <http://www.webmd.com/hypertension-high-blood-pressure/angiotensin-ii-receptor-blockers-arbs-for-high-blood-pressure>

23. "ACE Inhibitors for High Blood Pressure: Types, Uses, Effects ... - WebMD." 2007. 31 Jul. 2016 <http://www.webmd.com/hypertension-high-blood-pressure/ace-inhibitors-for-high-blood-pressure>

24. "Yoga, Blood Pressure, and Health - Medical News Today." 2013. 31 Jul. 2016 <http://www.medicalnewstoday.com/articles/260699.php>

25. "Beta blockers - Mayo Clinic." 2014. 3 Aug. 2016 <http://www.mayoclinic.org/diseases-conditions/high-blood-pressure/in-depth/beta-blockers/art-20044522>

26. "Calcium Channel Blockers for High Blood Pressure: Types ... - WebMD." 2012. 3 Aug. 2016

<http://www.webmd.com/hypertension-high-blood-pressure/guide/treatment-calcium-channel>

27. "Calcium channel blockers - Mayo Clinic." 2014. 3 Aug. 2016 <http://www.mayoclinic.org/diseases-conditions/high-blood-pressure/in-depth/calcium-channel-blockers/art-20047605>

28. "Aldosterone Receptor Antagonists: Diuretics for Heart Failure - WebMD." 2007. 12 Aug. 2016 <http://www.webmd.com/heart-disease/heart-failure/aldosterone-receptor-antagonists-diuretics-for-heart-failure>

29. "Alpha blockers - Mayo Clinic." 2014. 12 Aug. 2016 <http://www.mayoclinic.org/diseases-conditions/high-blood-pressure/in-depth/alpha-blockers/art-20044214>

30. "High blood pressure (hypertension) - Mayo Clinic." 2014. 12 Aug. 2016 <http://www.mayoclinic.org/diseases-conditions/high-blood-pressure/in-depth/high-blood-pressure-medication/art-20044451?pg=2>

31. "Vitamin D and hypertension | Vitamin D Council." 2013. 13 Aug. 2016 <https://www.vitamindcouncil.org/health-conditions/hypertension/>

32. "Herbs and Supplements for Hypertension ... - Everyday Health." 2009. 13 Aug. 2016 <http://www.everydayhealth.com/hypertension/herbs-and-supplements-for-hypertension.aspx>

33. "Coenzyme Q10 | University of Maryland Medical Center." 2013. 13 Aug. 2016 <http://umm.edu/health/medical/altmed/supplement/coenzyme-q10>

34. "Lowering Blood Pressure With Targeted Nutrients - Dr. David Williams." 2012. 13 Aug. 2016 <http://www.drdavidwilliams.com/blood-pressure-lowering-nutrients/>

35. "Magnesium Benefits Your Blood Pressure - Mercola." 2009. 13 Aug. 2016 <http://articles.mercola.com/sites/articles/archive/2009/06/11/magnesium-benefits-your-blood-pressure.aspx>

36. "Vitamin E & High Blood Pressure | LIVESTRONG.COM." 2010. 13 Aug. 2016 <http://www.livestrong.com/article/301209-vitamin-e-high-blood-pressure/>

37. "Low blood pressure (hypotension) Treatments and drugs - Mayo Clinic." 2014. 13 Aug. 2016 <http://www.mayoclinic.org/diseases-conditions/low-blood-pressure/basics/treatment/con-20032298>

38. "Tricks for everyday life with hypotension - Blood pressure and Tensoval." 2012. 13 Aug. 2016 <http://tensoval.com/tricks-for-everyday-life-with-hypotension.php>

39. "The Effects of Yoga on High Blood Pressure | Radiance Yoga." 2013. 15 Aug. 2016 <http://radiance-yoga.net/yoga-blood-pressure/>

40. "5 Poses to Reduce Hypertension | Yoga International." 2013. 15 Aug. 2016 <https://yogainternational.com/article/view/5-poses-to-reduce-hypertension>

41. "How to Do Bridge Pose in Yoga - YogaOutlet.com." 2016. 15 Aug. 2016 <https://www.yogaoutlet.com/guides/how-to-do-bridge-pose-in-yoga>

42. "How to Do Bridge Pose in Yoga - YogaOutlet.com." 2016. 15 Aug. 2016 <https://www.yogaoutlet.com/guides/how-to-do-bridge-pose-in-yoga>

43. "How to Do Hero Pose in Yoga - YogaOutlet.com." 2016. 15 Aug. 2016 <https://www.yogaoutlet.com/guides/how-to-do-hero-pose-in-yoga>

44. "Yoga for High Blood Pressure - Yoga Journal." 2014. 15 Aug. 2016 <http://www.yogajournal.com/category/poses/yoga-by-benefit/high-blood-pressure/>

45. "How to Do Corpse Pose in Yoga - YogaOutlet.com." 2016. 15 Aug. 2016 <https://www.yogaoutlet.com/guides/how-to-do-corpse-pose-in-yoga>

46. "Legs-Up-the-Wall Pose | Viparita Karani | Yoga Pose - Yoga Journal." 2014. 15 Aug. 2016 <http://www.yogajournal.com/pose/legs-up-the-wall-pose/>

47. "Yoga and High Blood Pressure - The American Yoga Association." 2006. 15 Aug. 2016 <http://www.americanyogaassociation.org/13hypertension.html>

48. "Low Blood Pressure Diagnosis & Treatment - WebMD." 2007. 16 Aug. 2016 <http://www.webmd.com/heart/understanding-low-blood-pressure-treatment>

Thank you again for downloading this book!

I hope this book was able to help you to gain a deeper understanding what blood pressure actually is and how you can improve it, with or without medication.

The next step is to take control and enjoy a healthy lifestyle.

Finally, if you enjoyed this book, then I'd like to ask you for a favor, would you be kind enough to leave a review for this book on Amazon? It'd be greatly appreciated!

If you want to be able to monitor your blood pressure affectively with an Amazon best selling blood pressure monitor, check out our product on Amazon:

<u>Blood pressure monitor with free carry case and UK adapter</u>

Thank you and good luck!

Preview of 'Meditation for Beginners'

Introduction

Welcome to the wonderful world of Meditation

You have obviously chosen to purchase this book for a reason. You are curious about meditation and you want to see what all of the fuss is about. A friend might have told you that they use mediation as a means of relaxation. Or else someone told you they use mediation to reach a "higher state of consciousness." You might be curious to see if meditation can help you with your daily life.

Then you have come to the right place, my friend. This book will give you a detailed guide into the art of mediation. We will discuss its history and origins as well as its true meaning. We will dispel some of the common "myths" and stereotypes regarding mediation. We will also tell you why meditation is beneficial to your overall health and well being.

We will give you different techniques for mediation and hints to help you get yourself into a daily routine. We will advise you on ways you can overcome obstacles that might prevent you from meditating on a daily basis.

We will discuss how mediation can raise your conscience and your mindfulness, as well as how it can reduce stress. Meditation can change your life in so many ways.

You might also be wondering what are the differences between yoga and meditation. We will discuss both and tell you how they can work hand in hand to lead you to a happier, healthier state of being.

If you've purchased this book, you are definitely intrigued by the concept of mediation. It is obviously more than just a curiosity by now. We can give you everything you need to know about the proper way to meditate.

Everyday life can be extremely stressful. Mediation can help ease your stress while relaxing your body, mind and soul.

What if meditation is against my religious beliefs?

There are many today, that are against the practice of meditation as they believe it opens the mind to another dimension and goes against the teachings of many religions. However, this is not the case. Most forms of religion use some form of mediation in their prayer or rituals, so do not let this discourage you. We will discuss how meditation is used in the various religions later on, but do not let anyone tell you that mediation is evil. Read the book in its entirety and then you can decide for yourself whether or not meditation goes against your personal beliefs. We are pretty sure you will be fairly surprised. Read on, my friends.

Stress and Anxiety

Life in today's high-tech, fast-paced, demanding society can be extremely overwhelming. You may often feel stressed and anxious. You might not be eating or sleeping properly. You feel as though you are constantly on edge. Did you know that stress is one of the leading causes of many health problems?

There are many factors in our lives that can cause us stress. Work, health, family issues, relationships, and the basic struggles of everyday life. Stress can cause immediate short-term effects such as rapid-breathing, sweaty palms, tightness in the chest and tension headaches. But if not treated properly, stress can lead to serious health issues.

Stress can lead to high blood pressure, heart disease, gastrointestinal disorders, autoimmune illnesses, mental issue and sleep disorders, among others. It is important to handle stress is a positive manner and find healthy ways to relieve stress so you can lead a happy and healthy life. It doesn't mean your problems will disappear, but you will be able to cope with them better.

How Meditation Can Help Reduce Stress

As we delve into the book, we will discuss exactly how meditation can help eliminate stress. To put it briefly, mediation can help relax your mind and your body. A simple ten-minute breathing meditation technique can help slow your heart rate and calm your racing thoughts. Meditating when your first awaken in the morning can help keep you relaxed and calm as you face your day. It can help clear your mind so you can better focus on the day ahead. Meditation before sleeping can help clear your mind and relax your body so you can have a restful sleep.

Benefits of Meditation

There are many advantages of meditation. We will discuss them in detail further on, but here are just a few to give you a general idea of how meditation can benefit your lifestyle.

Helps lower blood pressure

Assists in improving the immune system
Decreases anxiety
Sharpens the mind
Induces relaxation
Increases creativity
Boosts overall mood
Promotes happiness
Decrease pain levels
Boosts energy levels

There are many other benefits of meditation, which we will discuss later, but this give you a general idea of why meditation is so important in everyday life.

Types of Meditation

There are many types and techniques for mediation, whether you are a beginner or more experienced. We will discuss the techniques in great detail later in the book, but here are just a few different types of meditation to give you a general idea.

General Types of Meditation

Buddhist Meditation

Hindu Meditation
Chinese Meditation
Christian Meditation
Guided Meditation

Most Popular Meditation Techniques
Transcendental Meditation
Mindfulness Meditation
Chakra Meditation (Yoga)
Metta Meditation
Mantra Meditation
Zen Meditation

Again, these techniques, as well as others, will be discussed in great detail, we will tell you everything you need to know.

Mindfulness Meditation and Loving Kindness Meditation are two very simple forms of meditation that you can incorporate into your everyday life. Mindfulness Meditation can help you focus on the "here and now" and is a great way to fight anxiety and increase your focus. We have devoted an entire chapter to Mindfulness Meditation so you can have a better understanding as to how this type of meditation can benefit your everyday life.

Meditation is not complicated. Anyone can do it. Whether you take a few minutes to start your day or you want to take part a more involved routine, meditation can become an integral part of your everyday life.

So stick around. We are glad you decided to buy our meditation guide. Let us begin a journey together that can change your life for the better.

Click here to check out the rest of 'Meditation for Beginners' on Amazon.

Check Out Our Recommended Books:

Below you'll find some other popular books that are popular on Amazon and useful in reducing blood pressure and addressing issues that may affect blood pressure. Simply click on the links below to check them out.

Mindfulness
Meditation for Beginners
Anxiety Workbook
Reflexology: The Complete Guidebook

If the links do not work, for whatever reason, you can simply search for these titles on the Amazon website to find them.

Made in the USA
Lexington, KY
05 January 2017